DIABETES MELLITUS.

ALL YOU NEED TO KNOW ABOUT DIABETES MELLITUS.

TABLE OF CONTENTS.

WHAT IS DIABETES MELLITUS.

Diabetes Mellitus formally known as diabetes is one of the most common chronic diseases in the world. It is a common endocrine diseases characterized by sustained high blood sugar levels and a serious condition where your blood glucose level is too high.

It maybe or is a metabolic disease marked by high blood glucose, also known as blood sugar

Diabetes can also be the constant ailment that influences the body and transforms food into energy. The majority of the food you eat is separated into sugar (additionally called glucose) and delivered into your circulatory system. At the point when your glucose rises, then immediately it flags your pancreas to deliver insulin. Diabetes occurs when your body does not process food as energy properly. Insulin is a critical hormone that gets glucose (sugar that is used as energy) to the cells in your body. When you have diabetes, your body either doesn't respond to insulin or doesn't produce insulin at all. This causes sugars to build up in your blood, which puts you at risk of dangerous complications. Cell intake glucose from the bloodstream with the help of insulin. Glucose further breakdown in the cell process known as metabolism to generate ATP. ... Type-1 Diabetes is an autoimmune disease. Our own immune system attack the pancreatic cell which synthesizes insulin. Due to insulin formation decrease and body become resistant to glucose. Diabetes is a disease in which your body either can't produce insulin or can't properly use the insulin it produces. ... The importance of insulin. Diabetes is a disease in which your body either can't produce insulin or can't properly use the insulin it produces. Insulin is a hormone produced by your pancreas. Insulin's role is to regulate the amount of glucose (sugar) in the blood.

Diabetes can be understood in different ways and in other to better understand what diabetes is and how to treat it, it helps to learn about how the body works. Glucose: The Body's Fuel. The body is made up of millions of cells, and every cell needs energy. Your body uses glucose, or sugar, for energy. You need some glucose in your body at all times to live, even while you sleep.

Glucose is the fuel your body uses for energy. Diabetes is a major cause of morbidity and mortality, though these outcomes are not due to the immediate effects of the disorder. They are instead related to the diseases that develop as a result of chronic diabetes mellitus.

Certainly Diabetes is a long life condition.

TYPES OF DIABETES.

While there are different types of diabetes, they all stem from the body's inability to regulate blood sugar. Diabetes is caused by either a lack of insulin-secreting beta-cells in the pancreas due to an autoimmune response (type 1 diabetes), an imbalance between blood sugar level and insulin production (type 2 diabetes).

- Type 1 or Insulin Dependent Diabetes.

- Type 2 or non-insulin dependent diabetes

- Gestational or pregnancy period diabetes.

Type 1 diabetes: This type of diabetes is also known as Juvenile or Insulin Dependent Diabetes.

Diabetes mellitus (DM) type 1 is an autoimmune disorder characterized by insulin deficiency resulting from progressive destruction of the insulin-producing β cells of the pancreas. This insulin deficiency leads to hyperglycemia and ketosis. Chronic hyperglycemia is associated with long-term damage, leading to dysfunction of the kidney, eyes, nerves, heart, and blood vessels. In this condition, the pancreas makes little or no insulin. It is a metabolic disorder characterized by hyperglycemia due to absolute insulin deficiency. Patients most often present with a few days or weeks of polyuria, polydipsia, weight loss, and weakness. Some patients may present with diabetic ketoacidosis.It usually develops in children, teens, and young adults, but it can happen at any age. ... Diet and lifestyle habits don't cause type 1 diabetes. Type 1 diabetes occurs at every age and in people of every race, shape, and size.

Insulin is a hormone the body uses to allow sugar (glucose) to enter cells to produce energy.

It is a multisystem disease with both biochemical and anatomic/structural consequences. It is a chronic disease of carbohydrate, fat, and protein metabolism caused by the lack of insulin, which results from the marked and progressive inability of the pancreas to secrete insulin because of autoimmune destruction of the beta cells.

Different factors, such as genetics and some viruses, may cause type 1 diabetes. Although type 1 diabetes usually appears during childhood or adolescence, it can develop in adults. Type 1 diabetes has no cure. Treatment is directed toward managing the amount of sugar in the blood using insulin, diet and lifestyle to prevent complications.

TYPE 2 DIABETES;

Type 2 diabetes also known as non-insulin dependent diabetes is a form of diabetes mellitus caused by insulin resistance that leads to high blood sugar. It is the most common type of diabetes.

It is a chronic problem in which blood glucose (sugar) can no longer be regulated. There are two reasons for this. First, the cells of the body become resistant to insulin (insulin resistant). Insulin works like a key to let glucose (blood sugar) move out of the blood and into the cells where it is used as fuel for energy. When the cells become insulin resistant, it requires more and more insulin to move sugar into the cells, and too much sugar stays in the blood. Over time, if the cells require more and more insulin, the pancreas can't make enough insulin to keep up and begins to fail. Type 2 diabetes is a form of diabetes mellitus caused by insulin resistance that leads to high blood sugar. . Type 2 diabetes mellitus is often associated with certain genetic predispositions, environmental factors, lifestyle choices, and the dynamic interactions between all of these different aspects. This ailment is a disease state which involves the dysfunction of insulin-producing pancreatic beta cells, insulin hormone resistance in cells of the body, or a combination of both. Diabetes mellitus type 2 is a condition that typically begins with resistance to insulin by cells of the body that worsens over time. This resistance, and the compensating production of insulin by pancreatic beta cells may eventually lead to beta cell failure. When the beta cells fail, endogenous insulin can no longer be secreted.

Insulin resistance is the inability of cells to use the insulin hormone, which inhibits the cell's capability to absorb and then use glucose in metabolic processes. This is of primary concern in cells that are typically high in metabolic function, such as muscle, liver, and adipose tissues. Since insulin is responsible for the cellular uptake of glucose, the sugar molecules will remain in the bloodstream.

The pancreatic beta cells, which are responsible for producing and releasing insulin, may also dysfunction in type 2 diabetes mellitus. If the insulin supply diminishes entirely, the individual will be dependent upon exogenous insulin.

Whether insulin is not present due to hyposecretion, or if the hormone is rendered useless because of insulin resistance, the end result will be hyperglycemia. Hyperglycemia, or elevated glucose levels within the blood, is the hallmark of type 2 diabetes mellitus. Hyperglycemia, and the associated inflammatory processes lead to the micro and macro-vascular changes that are seen as complications of diabetes mellitus.

GESTATIONAL DIABETES:

This is also known as Pregnancy period diabetes.Gestational diabetes is diabetes diagnosed for the first time during pregnancy (gestationGestational diabetes mellitus (GDM) is a condition in which a hormone made by the placenta prevents the body from using insulin effectively. Glucose builds up in the blood instead of being absorbed by the cells.

Unlike type 1 diabetes, gestational diabetes is not caused by a lack of insulin, but by other hormones produced during pregnancy that can make insulin less effective, a condition referred to as insulin resistance. Gestational diabetic symptoms disappear following delivery. Although the cause of GDM is not known, there are some theories as to why the condition occurs.

The placenta supplies a growing fetus with nutrients and water, and also produces a variety of hormones to maintain the pregnancy. Some of these hormones (estrogen, cortisol, and human placental lactogen) can have a blocking effect on insulin. This is called contra-insulin effect, which usually begins about 20 to 24 weeks into the pregnancy.

As the placenta grows, more of these hormones are produced, and the risk of insulin resistance becomes greater. Normally, the pancreas is able to make additional insulin to overcome insulin resistance, but when the production of insulin is not enough to overcome the effect of the placental hormones, gestational diabetes results.

DIAGNOSIS OF DIABETES.

The only way to know for sure that you have diabetes is to get tested. Blood tests that measure your blood glucose (sugar) levels. These can be arranged through your GP. A diagnosis of diabetes is always confirmed by laboratory results. The most common tests are the A1C test and the plasma glucose test.

- **A1C test.** This blood test, which doesn't require not eating for a period of time (fasting), shows your average blood sugar level for the past 2 to 3 months. It measures the percentage of blood sugar attached to hemoglobin, the oxygen-carrying protein in red blood cells. It's also called a glycated hemoglobin test.

The higher your blood sugar levels, the more hemoglobin

you'll have with sugar attached. An A1C level of 6.5% or higher on two separate tests means that you have diabetes. An A1C between 5.7% and 6.4% means that you have prediabetes. Below 5.7% is considered normal.

- **Random blood sugar test.** A blood sample will be taken at a random time. No matter when you last ate, a blood sugar level of 200 milligrams per deciliter (mg/dL) — 11.1 millimoles per liter (mmol/L) — or higher suggests diabetes.

- **Fasting blood sugar test.** A blood sample will be taken after you haven't eaten anything the night before (fast). A fasting blood sugar level less than 100 mg/dL (5.6 mmol/L) is normal. A fasting blood sugar level from 100 to 125 mg/dL (5.6 to 6.9 mmol/L) is considered prediabetes. If it's 126 mg/dL (7 mmol/L) or higher on two separate tests, you have diabetes.

- **Glucose tolerance test.** For this test, you fast overnight. Then, the fasting blood sugar level is measured. Then you drink a sugary liquid, and blood sugar levels are tested regularly for the next two hours.

A blood sugar level less than 140 mg/dL (7.8 mmol/L) is

normal. A reading of more than 200 mg/dL (11.1 mmol/L) after two hours means you have diabetes. A reading between 140 and 199 mg/dL (7.8 mmol/L and 11.0 mmol/L) means you have prediabetes.

If your provider thinks you may have type 1 diabetes, they may test your urine to look for the presence of ketones. Ketones are a byproduct produced when muscle and fat are used for energy. Your provider will also probably run a test to see if you have the destructive immune system cells associated with type 1 diabetes called autoantibodies.

Your provider will likely see if you're at high risk for gestational diabetes early in your pregnancy. If you're at high risk, your provider may test for diabetes at your first prenatal visit. If you're at average risk, you'll probably be screened sometime during your second trimester.

SIGNS AND SYMPTOMS OF DIABETES.

Often, there are no symptoms. When symptoms do occur, they include excessive thirst or urination, fatigue, weight loss or blurred vision.

Some of the symptoms of type 1 diabetes and type 2 diabetes are:

- Feeling more thirsty than usual.

- Urinating often.

- Losing weight without trying.

- Presence of ketones in the urine. Ketones are a byproduct of the breakdown of muscle and fat that happens when there's not enough available insulin.

- Feeling tired and weak.

- Feeling irritable or having other mood changes.

- Having blurry vision.

- Having slow-healing sores.

- Getting a lot of infections, such as gum, skin and vaginal infections.

Some of the symptoms of gestational diabetes are

Morning sickness

Fatigue

Lower abdominal pain few times.

CAUSES OF DIABETES.

There are no actual or specific of the many believed causes of Diabetes that has been proven scientifically.

- Type 1 diabetes occurs when your immune system, the body's system for fighting infection, attacks and destroys the insulin-producing beta cells of the pancreas. Scientists think type 1 diabetes is caused by genes and environmental factors, such as viruses, that might trigger the disease.

- Type 2 diabetes—the most common form of diabetes—is caused by several factors, including lifestyle factors and genes.

Overweight, obesity, and physical inactivity

Insulin resistance

Genes and family history

- Gestational diabetes is thought to arise because the many changes, hormonal and otherwise, that occur in the body during pregnancy predispose some women to become resistant to insulin. Insulin is a hormone made by specialized cells in the pancreas that allows the body to effectively metabolize glucose for later usage as fuel (energy). When levels of insulin are low, or the body cannot effectively use insulin (i.e., insulin resistance), blood glucose levels rise.

TREATMENT OF DIABETES.

People with diabetes benefit greatly from learning about the disorder, understanding how diet and exercise affect their blood glucose levels, and knowing how to avoid complications. A nurse trained in diabetes education can provide information about managing diet, exercising, monitoring blood glucose levels, and taking medication.

People with diabetes should stop smoking and consume only moderate amounts of alcohol (up to one drink per day for women and two for men).Diet, exercise, and education are the cornerstones of treatment of diabetes and often the first recommendations for people with mild diabetes. Weight loss is important for people who are overweight. People who continue to have elevated blood glucose levels despite lifestyle changes, or have very high blood glucose levels and people with type 1 diabetes (no matter their blood glucose levels) also require medication.

Because complications are less likely to develop if people with diabetes strictly control their blood glucose levels, the goal of diabetes treatment is to keep blood glucose levels as close to the normal range as possible.

It is helpful for people with diabetes to carry or wear medical identification (such as a bracelet or tag) to alert health care practitioners to the presence of diabetes. This information allows health care practitioners to start life-saving treatment quickly, especially in the case of injury or change in mental status.

- Diet

Diet management is very important in people with either type of diabetes mellitus. Doctors recommend a healthy, balanced diet and efforts to maintain a healthy weight. People with diabetes can benefit from meeting with a dietitian or a diabetes educator to develop an optimal eating plan. Such a plan includes

Avoiding simple sugars and processed foods

Increasing dietary fiber

Limiting portions of carbohydrate-rich and fatty foods (especially saturated fats)

People who are taking insulin should avoid long periods between meals to prevent hypoglycemia. Although protein and fat in the diet contribute to the number of calories a person eats, only the number of carbohydrates has a direct effect on blood glucose levels. The American Diabetes Association has many helpful tips on diet, including recipes.

Even when people follow a proper diet, cholesterol-lowering medication are often needed to decrease the risk of heart disease.

People with type 1 diabetes and certain people with type 2 diabetes may use carbohydrate counting or the carbohydrate exchange system to match their insulin dose to the carbohydrate content of their meal. "Counting" the amount of carbohydrate in a meal is used to calculate the amount of insulin the person takes before eating. However, the carbohydrate-to-insulin ratio (the amount of insulin taken for each gram of carbohydrate in the meal) varies for each person, and people with diabetes need to work closely with a dietician who has experience in working with people with diabetes to master the technique. Some experts have advised use of the glycemic index (a measure of the impact of an ingested carbohydrate-containing food on the blood glucose level) to delineate between rapid and slowly metabolized carbohydrates, although there is little evidence to support this approach.

- Exercise

Exercise, in appropriate amounts (at least 150 minutes a week spread out over at least three days), can also help people control their weight and improve blood glucose levels. Because blood glucose levels go down during exercise, people must be alert for symptoms of hypoglycemia. Some people need to eat a small snack during prolonged exercise, decrease their insulin dose, or both.

- Weight loss

Many people, especially those with type 2 diabetes, are overweight or obese. Some people with type 2 diabetes may be able to avoid or delay the need to take medications by achieving and maintaining a healthy weight. Weight loss is also important in these people because excess weight contributes to complications of diabetes. When obese people with diabetes have trouble losing weight with diet and exercise alone, doctors may give weight-loss medication or recommend bariatric surgery (surgery to cause weight loss). Certain diabetes medications can induce weight loss, especially glucagon-like peptide 1 (GLP-1) and SGLT2 inhibitor medications.

Sometimes a doctor will recommend a medication that helps with weight loss.

- Pancreas transplantation

People with type 1 diabetes sometimes receive transplantation of an entire pancreas or of only the insulin-producing cells from a donor pancreas. This procedure may allow people with type 1 diabetes mellitus to maintain normal glucose levels. However, because immunosuppressant medications must be given to prevent the body from rejecting the transplanted cells, pancreas transplantation is usually done only in people who have serious complications due to diabetes or who are receiving another transplanted organ (such as a kidney) and will require immunosuppressants anyway.

Treatment for gestational diabetes involves attention to maintaining a proper diet. Nutritional modification is the mainstay of therapy, and many women will achieve adequate glucose control by following a nutritional plan. Regular exercise can also contribute to tight glucose control.

COMPLICATIONS OF DIABETES TREATMENT

- Poor vision, limited manual dexterity due to arthritis, tremor, or stroke, or other physical limitations may make monitoring blood glucose levels more difficult for some people. However, special monitors are available. Some have large numerical displays that are easier to read. Some provide audible instructions and results. Some monitors read blood glucose levels through the skin and do not require a blood sample. People can consult a diabetes educator to determine which meter is most appropriate.

- Hypoglycemia

The most common complication of treating high blood

glucose levels is low blood glucose levels (hypoglycemia). The risk is greatest for people who are frail, who are sick enough to require frequent hospital admissions, or who are taking several medications. Of all available medications to treat diabetes, long-acting sulfonylurea medications or insulin are most likely to cause low blood glucose levels in people with severe or many medical problems and especially in older people. When they take these medications, these people are also more likely to have serious symptoms, such as fainting and falling, and to have difficulty thinking or using parts of the body due to low blood glucose levels.

In older people, hypoglycemia may be less obvious than in younger people. Confusion caused by hypoglycemia may be mistaken for dementia or the sedative effect of medications. Also, people who have difficulty communicating (as after a stroke or as a result of dementia) may not be able to let anyone know they are having symptoms.

RISK FACTORS OF DIABETES.

These are factors that easily predispose one or increases the chances of diabetes of a person.

Type 1

This type usually starts in childhood. Your pancreas stops making insulin. You have type 1 diabetes for life. The main things that lead to it are:

- Family history. If you have relatives with diabetes, chances are higher that you'll get it, too. Anyone who has a mother, father, sister, or brother with type 1 diabetes should get checked. A simple blood test can diagnose it.

- Diseasess of the pancreas. They can slow its ability to make insulin.

- Infection or illness. Some infections and illnesses, mostly rare ones, can damage your pancreas.

Type 2

If you have this kind, your body can't use the insulin it makes. This is called insulin resistance. Type 2 usually affects adults, but it can begin at any time in your life. The main things that lead to it are

- Obesity or being overweight. Research shows this is a top reason for type 2 diabetes. Because of the rise in obesity among U.S. children, this type is affecting more teenagers.

- Impaired glucose tolerance. Prediabetes is a milder form of this condition. It can be diagnosed with a simple blood test. If you have it, there's a strong chance you'll get type 2 diabetes.

- Insulin resistance. Type 2 diabetes often starts with cells that are resistant to insulin. That means your pancreas has to work extra hard to make enough insulin to meet your body's needs.

- Ethnic background. Diabetes happens more often in Hispanic/Latino Americans, African-Americans, Native Americans, Asian-Americans, Pacific Islanders, and Alaska natives.

- Gestational diabetes. If you had diabetes while you were pregnant, you had gestational diabetes. This raises your chances of getting type 2 diabetes later in life.

- Sedentary lifestyle. You exercise less than three times a week.

- Family history. You have a parent or sibling who has diabetes.

- Polycystic ovary syndrome. Women with polycystic ovary syndrome (PCOS) have a higher risk.

- Age. If you're over 45 and overweight or if you have symptoms of diabetes, talk to your doctor about a simple screening test.

Gestational Diabetes.

It's caused by hormones the placenta makes or by too little insulin. High blood sugar from the mother causes high blood sugar in the baby. That can lead to growth and development problems if left untreated. Things that can lead to gestational diabetes include:

- Obesity or being overweight. Extra pounds can lead to gestational diabetes.

- Glucose intolerance. Having glucose intolerance or gestational diabetes in the past makes you more likely to get it again.

- Family history. If a parent or sibling has had gestational diabetes, you're more likely to get it.

- Age. The older you are when you get pregnant, the higher your chances are.

- Ethnic background. Nonwhite women have a greater chance of developing it.

Complications of Diabetes Mellitus.

- Diabetes long-term consequences emerge gradually. The risk of problems increases with the duration of diabetes and the degree to which your blood sugar is under control. Diabetes problems could eventually become incapacitating or even fatal. In actuality, type 2 diabetes can result from prediabetes. Potential issues include:

- cardiovascular disease (heart and blood vessel disease). Diabetes significantly raises the risk of numerous heart conditions. They include heart attacks, strokes, arterial narrowing, and coronary artery disease with chest pain (angina) (atherosclerosis). Diabetes increases your risk of developing heart disease or stroke.

- diabetic nerve injury (diabetic neuropathy). The walls of the tiny blood arteries (capillaries) that feed the nerves might become damaged by an excessive sugar intake, especially in the legs. The tingling, numbness, burning, or pain that may result from this typically starts at the tips of the toes or fingers and progressively moves higher.

- Problems with nausea, vomiting, diarrhea, or constipation can result from damage to the nerves that control digestion. It might cause erectile dysfunction in men.

- Diabetes can cause kidney damage (diabetic nephropathy). The glomeruli, which are millions of microscopic blood artery clusters in the kidneys, filter the blood's waste. This delicate filtering system can be harmed by diabetes.

- diabetes's impact on the eyes (diabetic retinopathy). The blood vessels in the eyes might get damaged by diabetes. Blindness could result from this.

- Foot injury. Many foot issues are made more likely by nerve injury in the feet or inadequate blood circulation to the feet.

- oral and skin ailments. You may be more vulnerable to bacterial and fungal infections as a result of diabetes.

- impairment of hearing. Diabetes patients are more likely to experience hearing issues.

- Alzheimer's condition. Alzheimer's disease and other forms of dementia may be more likely in people with type 2 diabetes.

diabetes-related depression. Diabetes patients of both types 1 and type 2 frequently experience depressive symptoms.

gestational diabetes complications

Pregnant mothers with gestational diabetes typically have healthy births. Untreated or unmanaged blood sugar levels, however, can harm both you and your unborn child.

Pregnancy complications brought on by gestational diabetes include:

- excessive expansion. The placenta can allow more glucose to pass. The baby's pancreas produces more insulin in response to increased glucose. Your baby can become too big as a result of this. It may result in a challenging delivery and occasionally necessitate a C-section.

- low sugar levels. Shortly after birth, newborns of gestational diabetic moms can experience low blood sugar (hypoglycemia). They produce a lot of insulin on their own, which explains this.

- diabetes type 2 later in life. Infants whose mothers with gestational diabetes are more likely to grow up obese and develop type 2 diabetes.

- Death. Uncontrolled gestational diabetes increases the risk of a baby's death either during pregnancy or soon after birth.

Gestational diabetes can potentially result in maternal complications, such as:

- Preeclampsia. High blood pressure, an excessive amount of protein in the urine, and swelling in the legs and feet are all signs of this illness.

- pregnancy diabetes. You are more likely to develop gestational diabetes again if you already had it during one pregnancy.

PREVENTION OF DIABETES MELLITUS.

Diabetes type 1 cannot be stopped. Yet, adopting a healthy lifestyle may help avoid gestational diabetes, type 2 diabetes, and prediabetes as well as treat them.

- Consume nutritious meals. Choose meals with more fiber and less calories and fat. Put an emphasis on whole grains, veggies, and fruits. Consume a variety of foods to avoid becoming bored.

- Start moving more often. On most days of the week, try to engage in around 30 minutes of moderate aerobic exercise. Alternatively try to do 150 minutes or more of moderate aerobic exercise each week. Take a brisk daily stroll as an example. Break up a lengthy exercise into shorter periods throughout the day if you are unable to fit it in.

- Lose any extra weight. If you are overweight, even a 7% weight loss may reduce your chance of developing diabetes. If you weigh 200 pounds (90.7 kilograms), for instance, decreasing 14 pounds (6.4 kilograms) may reduce your chance of developing diabetes.

Therefore, avoid attempting to reduce weight when pregnant.
Find out from your doctor how much weight you may safely
acquire while expecting.

- Work on long-term improvements to your food and
  exercise routines to maintain a healthy weight.
  Keep in mind the advantages of decreasing weight,
  like a healthier heart, increased energy, and
  improved self-esteem.

- Drugs are a possibility on occasion. Type 2 diabetes
  risk may be decreased by oral diabetic medications
  like metformin (Glumetza, Fortamet, and others).
  Nonetheless, adopting a healthy lifestyle is crucial.
  Check your blood sugar at least once a year if you
  have prediabetes to ensure sure type 2 diabetes has
  not yet manifested.